POWER WALKING – HOW TO BURN BELLY FAT BY WALKING 10,000 STEPS (& EATING POWERFUL NUTRIENTS)

Introduction

When it comes to power walking it's reassuring to know that your long-term success will be gained in a short period of time just by perseverance. You will be able to drop those unwanted pounds from the midsection, gain a great metabolism that won't let you down and build lean muscle, all from power walking. This book will also give you food tips on the best nutrients that will optimise your hard work, and make sure you get the most out of it. Not only this, but anxiety and stress will be relieved due to your body's natural endorphins that are released as your serotonin levels are boosted by your efforts. All you need to do, is take those first steps and you'll find that it is not willpower driving you but rather 'want power' pulling you towards your goal.

Let's Achieve Those Goals

In order to achieve our goals, we first need to know what they are. This is vital in order for us to succeed, so we can be realistic about the weight we want to be and set our expectations accordingly. So instead of being unrealistic, let's set achievable goals that will not only allow you to drop pounds from your waist, but also improve your overall health and eating habits. Your goals don't have to be amazingly complex, as long as you're specific about how you visualise your long-term result. For example, they could be increasing your muscle mass, dropping pounds and then maintaining the body shape you desire, or lowering your blood pressure. Instead of being short sporadic efforts that do not have longevity, these efforts require gradual and sustainable changes to your life habits.

Significant Milestones

If you set yourself small milestones to achieve, as you achieve them they will bring you a step closer to your desired result, and allow you to reach your goal. So, dropping 10 pounds can be a small milestone that will bring you closer to your end goal of maintaining a lower body weight - just make sure you give yourself time to achieve this. As you go along, your strength and endurance will increase and then you will be able to re-evaluate your small milestones to make your workouts more intense and even more rewarding. For example, walking further distances and walking with small hand weights will burn the fat a lot more quickly.

What You Need For Success

A vital part in helping you achieve weight loss by walking, is having the correct equipment for your workouts. Comfortable walking shoes that provide good arch support, a multi-functioning pedometer and a journal to record your achievements are all important. Realistically, you will need to build up to walking 10,000 steps per day. So a good thing to do is create realistic small milestones that will bring you closer to that 10,000 steps per day. Mark down in your journal the small achievements as you achieve them because this will give you a great feeling of accomplishment.

How To Use Positive Reinforcement

When you see changes in yourself, your body and your weight, mark them down in your journal especially when they are unexpected.

Some great changes that you may notice could be increased muscle tone, feeling less stressed, getting a better night's sleep, or feeling younger. Whatever they are, marking them down and acknowledging them will benefit you greatly and increase your commitment levels.

The Positive Effects of Walking

There are many benefits of walking for weight loss that many of us at first don't realise. When you see these changes and take note of them you are much more likely to stick with it, because you see how walking can really alter your body shape and boost your health. Power walking is a great form of cardiovascular exercise and strength training combined, and is low-impact on the body and joints. Other health benefits are keeping age-related diseases away, reduced belly fat, reducing your stress or anxiety, deterring heart disease and dropping pounds. Although walking for weight loss is designed to drop pounds, try to remember that your efforts are also changing your life and restructuring your life habits. By remembering this you can absolutely stay proactive and positive in striving to reach your milestones, and this is a great mind-set to have.

How To Optimise Fat Burning By Power Walking

Although it may be tempting to progress from walking to jogging or running, these exercises can actually be more detrimental because they can directly affect your knees and joints due to the way you bounce off the floor as you jog or run. Power walking is a much better alternative and here's why: it has great benefits such as taking less time to burn off fat and calories, improved thought processes and improved brain functioning, but it is also a low-stress exercise

that is easy on your joints due to the gliding movement of the power walker. In next to no time you'll be looking better and there's no need to worry about getting injured whilst doing it.

Selecting The Right Footwear

Because power walking requires pushing your body harder than normal walking, it's important to have the right shoes. It's a little-known fact that power walkers actually walk the same speed as joggers, however joggers hit the floor with twice as much force. The body mechanics between the two are very different, as real progress in power walking is achieved by the walker pumping their arms, both engaging the abdomen and clenching the buttocks therefore gliding horizontally in a graceful motion. When done correctly, the abdomen remaining tense throughout the walk and this will ensure that it becomes toned and sheds pounds from the midsection.

So, select footwear that is both flexible and allows for good motion in the middle range of the foot by giving good arch support. To avoid strain in the heels and the shins stay away from flat and hard souls that don't have much flexibility. Because power walking requires long even strides, flexibility is key in selecting footwear for advanced walking.

When it comes to footwear it is also important to make sure that they are made with natural wicking materials. This will give you the ventilation when you sweat, and you should be aware that shoes you need for power walking is quite different to the shoes that you need for jogging or running.

To avoid chaffing and unwanted friction when power walking it is very important that you select the appropriate pants that are both comfortable and flexible. Most tracksuit bottoms or work-out pants will be fine for power walking, and as you build-up speed you make sure that they remain comfortable.

Before You Set Out

Take a little bit of time to gradually build up to a good pace rather than just setting out at your fastest speed as it usually takes about 5 to 10 minutes to get your muscles fully warmed up. So, after a couple of minutes stop and stretch your shoulders, arms and hamstrings, then while keeping your hips still stretch your waist by bending the upper torso to each side. Unlike normal walking, power walking is absolutely a full body exercise therefore you should stretch from your head all the way down to your toes before you embark on the main portion of your walk.

Total Body Conditioning

The major muscle groups become toned and firmed up during this type of walking because it requires people to use all of their muscles. To burn the maximum amount of fat and calories when power walking, always engage your core muscles. You can do this by imagining there is a string attached to your midsection and someone who is taller than you is standing behind you and pulling the string thereby drawing your stomach up and back. So when you draw your navel up and in, your core muscles will be totally engaged throughout your walk. Keep this up for the duration of your power

walk, and you'll see major changes in the conditioning and toning of your stomach.

Like everything, this will become easier as time goes on, as when you first try it it may be hard to keep your abs engaged the whole time. The muscles at the sides of your torso (your obliques), will be engaged by your opposite arm and leg movements while you walk, so the combined motion of your limbs as you stride will give your torso good muscle tone.

As well as focusing on your abs, make sure your buttocks are engaged for the duration of the walk. The combination of tightening up your abs and buttocks is what turns this cardio exercise into a genuine strength training exercise, which results in maximising the amount of calories you burn. Lean muscle will be developed even when walking horizontally across a flat plain as your body burns calories, and therefore you will see a dramatic increase in your metabolism.

Why You Should Walk 4.5 Miles Per Hour

Not dissimilar to the speed of jogging, the target speed of 4.5 mph is perfect for power walking. Try to make sure your strides are long and even and focus on matching your leg movements with your arm movements, as when performed properly there should be a slight but easy sway to your hips. This will allow you to reach greater speeds with ease, but make sure this doesn't break into a slow run. This is because when you jog or run you are performing both vertical and horizontal movements, and when you're power walking you should only be striding horizontally, not bouncing off the ground at

all. If you find yourself doing this, just slow down a little bit and adjust your stride accordingly because maintaining good form is very beneficial when it comes to shedding pounds from walking.

When walking at a moderate and slow pace it is rare to feel out of breath or break a sweat, due to it being a moderate impact activity. And although it can burn a lot of calories and get rid of fat it doesn't have much effect on your respiratory system or cardio. But when you up the ante to power walking, the first few times it's normal to feel knackered and winded. So during the first few times you power walk listen to your body and pay attention to how it feels now that you have boosted your walking speed. Think about how your shoes feel and think about which areas of your body are struggling, and if your hips start to ache you could always take the activity to a shock absorbing surface like a track. Your ankles and knees should feel fine if you're power walking correctly, but your hips may start to hurt when you first attempt it and that is when you can possibly try a different surface.

How To Reach Faster Speeds Consistently

This is the easiest way to work out your speed: know how far you're walking and how long it takes to get there, then divide the walking distance by the number of hours that it takes you to walk this far and this will equal the number of miles per hour you are travelling. So, from the outset try to walk for one full hour, and due to the moderate impact of the exercise you're not likely to experience any injury or bodily stress.

To get your speed up, the best way is to pump your arms harder and faster, because then your legs will follow. The reason why you use your arms to gain speed is because if you focus on your legs then your buttocks may begin to experience a burning sensation. You may not need to train for a full hour given that you can burn more calories in less time with power walking. But if you can manage it, you get a lot more benefits such as a greater release of endorphins and a greater amount of stress relief as well as emotional, physical and mental benefits. It's easier to walk for longer than jog or run because of the relative ease of this activity even if the exercise is pretty new to you. You could always stop for a moment to get your breath back and then go harder once to energy has regained.

To get to the 4.5 per hour pace, you need to build up to it as this means you will be power walking a whole mile in about 30 min which isn't going to be easy straightaway. So, instead of trying to go to full-on and then burning out after a few minutes, pushing your body to go longer while simultaneously using the correct form will give you way better results. Because at a speed of about 4.5 mph you can burn off just over 200 calories in only half an hour, and this can be better than jogging because you're using the same amount of energy either way. You'll notice great improvements in your target speed by holding a small pair of handheld weights or by strapping on some ankle weights, as this will push you way beyond just improving the speed of your walking. There are also benefits of doing this exercise indoors if the weather is bad, such as using a treadmill because it will give you the option of altering the incline of the walking service to increase the challenge therefore burning more calories.

Why You Shouldn't Always Walk At Your Fastest Pace

When walking for an entire hour, the best way to minimise your risk of physical injury is a power walking plan where you can gradually increase in speed, with a period of peak speed and then gradually slow down at the end. You shouldn't come to a sudden standstill at the end of the hour, and you shouldn't start out with big quick strides. So, at the end of the exercise spend at least 10 minutes bringing your body back down to a steady pace slowly. Your breathing should return to normal and your heart should be beating slowly by the time you have stopped walking. When you're ready for your post-workout stretching, your muscles will be feeling warm and ready for it. You should focus on doing the same stretch routine you did during the warm-up, but make sure you add in your abs and buttocks as this will give you the whole body post-workout stretch routine that you need.

The Psychological Benefits of Power Walking

When walking at optimal speeds, not only will your body reward you for your efforts but your brain will too. Benefits include de-cluttering your mind, de-stressing, and giving you a stimulating rush of endorphins. Indeed, you will also have increased levels of inner calm and peace as this activity allows for introspection Studies have shown that regular walking improves sleep and helps to slow mental decline considerably. It also helps by focussing on breathing and other basic and automatic functions whilst clearing the brain of external stressors as it is the ideal opportunity to operate with meditative intent. So, if dropping pounds isn't enough motivation for

you, think about your overall well-being, less anxiety or depression and having a far greater energy as benefits worth aiming for.

Nutrition and Power Walking - What You Should Eat and Why

It is absolutely possible to shed pounds in just the first couple of weeks of power walking, as it is a great combination of both strength training and cardio exercise, so you'll be able to visually see the difference in your body. But if you want to really make the most of your hard work and optimise your results, you can add a good diet plan. So work to fuel your body with a great array of powerful nutrients instead of completely focusing on cutting calories alone. Here's how.

The Best Foods

You'll be building new lean muscle from power walking and if you need a bit of extra fuel your metabolism can burn off more fat and calories. This can easily be done with strength training. Foods with a lot of protein will always be the best thing to consume if you want to increase lean muscle because protein is the only thing the builds lean muscle. Carbs and fats are energy sources whereas protein is vital in increasing your metabolism and maintaining lean muscle. So feed your body what it needs to regenerate and rebuild the targeted muscle groups after a power walking routine by eating the right high protein foods. Natural food sources are always the best way to go when getting essential nutrients, and this is preferable above supplements that some people rely on. This is because the body finds it easier to break down and recognise protein in this form –

even some of the highest quality supplements won't be fully be absorbed by the body and what the body can't use it just get rid of.

As well as the obvious choices of white meat, fish and other animal derived protein, there is also the great option of true nuts such as walnuts, pecans and almonds as these are optimal sources of protein. Almond butter and nut butters are also optimal sources of protein, but steer clear of peanuts as they are not a true nut and are packed with way more starch so will be detrimental to your walking for weight loss goal.

Other good sources of protein are chickpeas, lentils, pinto beans, kidney beans, red beans, and black beans as these are low in fat and high in protein. They can easily be made into a tasty soup and other dishes to power up after a workout and replenish your body. They are also easy on the wallet and due to them being very high in protein they are also rich in magnesium, fibre, iron and potassium. They increase and improve your digestive regularity, improve your heart health and they can increase your collagen production. So by adding these to your diet you can avoid many health risks whilst simultaneously building muscle. By improving your diet with their protein dense nature you will also reduce the risk of physical injury. They are also very filling so there's not much chance of going hungry and lacking energy.

The best meats when it comes to protein is white meats such as fish, chicken and turkey breast because they are full of nutrients and can be a good base for soups, pasta and salad. Several servings per week will help you gain lean muscle but be careful of your fish supplier due to increased mercury levels.

Which Foods Will Give You The Most Energy

The most essential foods for maintaining a high level of energy when power walking are carbohydrates. When selecting the right carbohydrates, be aware of the huge difference between natural sources of carbohydrates that give the body energy and nourishment versus those that are heavily refined. These have a bad reputation due to the major weight gain that is possible by consuming too much of them.

Other sources of fuel that are good can come in the form of vegetables and fresh fruits as these are water dense, are rich in nourishment, rich in vitamins and overall are low in calories. When maintaining your walking for weight loss exercise plan, minimising the amount of empty calorie foods you consume is vital. This is because these foods have been stripped of almost all of their nutritional benefits. White flour is one example to stay away from, because when consumed these carbs are converted into sugars in no time, and therefore can be detrimental to your internal organ systems as well as increasing your risk of other nutrition related health problems. When it comes to grains, products that are offered in the closest form of their natural state are the ones that you should always go for.

A good way to help regulate your blood sugar levels and get rid of bad toxins from your blood flow is to eat steel cut oatmeal. This decreases your risk of developing diabetes and adding cinnamon makes it tasty. Consuming hot oatmeal with chopped fruit such as blackberries, blueberries or any other unprocessed nutritional fruit will give a good boost to your health. You can also add nuts into this

mix, pecans being a good choice as they are able to provide the body with an added rich dose of protein. This kind of meal is really beneficial to the heart and one that will absolutely give you the energy that is needed to maintain a gruelling one hour power walking session.

A Well-Balanced Blend of Essential Food Groups Is Key

A lot of the reasons why people develop weight loss issues is by not sticking to good habits when it comes to eating. Some diet plans are also missing a lot of ingredients that require balance. There is good and bad fat - when people pursue too much of bad fat along with too many refined carbs it becomes a downward spiral to weight gain. And when they try to compensate by swinging in the opposite way, they often cut out major food groups like carbohydrates entirely. Carbohydrates are needed in order to represent a well-balanced blend of all the essential food groups. So instead of dropping pounds fast they are actually denying their bodies important powerful nutrients that will benefit them in their exercise regime.

Although cutting out carbohydrates entirely can absolutely help you drop pounds, these types of diets don't last long and the reason why is because as soon as the individual returns to their old eating habits, the lost weight will return rapidly. Cutting out carbohydrates entirely causes the metabolism to slow down, so it's always a good idea to give your body the nutrients it needs. Sticking to roughly 2000 calories per day will help you reach a healthy weight more quickly than anything else, and once there it will be far easier to maintain it.

Fresh Is Best

When snacking, the best way to reduce unwanted calories is to always eat fresh. You get a rush of natural energy by eating an apple as well as keeping your teeth clean, likewise a handful of sugar snow peas will give you three times the recommended daily amount of vitamin C that your body needs. So, absolutely stay clear of chips, cookies, cakes, and processed sandwich bread as these foods will contain an unhealthy amount of calories, sodium, sugar and fat and will provide no benefit to your body, so don't rely on them. Another benefit of vegetables and fresh fruits are that they are very dense in fibre as well as being filled with water, and this is important after a power walking regime as they will replenish your stores thereby minimising the amount of water that you need to drink in order to stay hydrated.

Good Oil and Bad Fats

It's a good idea to limit the amount of cream, cheese and butter you consume as part of your regular diet as these dairy products contain a lot of fat. Instead, get healthy fats from fish, olives and nuts. The best cooking oil is coconut due to its antibacterial properties as well as being able to be heated at high heats without chemically changing due to its stable nature. Try to avoid olive oil - even though it has the reputation of being the best oil for a healthy diet, it's actually highly unstable and the composition of its chemicals change once it is heated, so it's therefore greatly inferior to coconut oil. Cold it's fine though on salads, but avoid it when it comes to boiling of frying.

It's recommended that you should try to eat at least one full tablespoon of coconut oil per day as this will be of great benefit to your diet. It has vital nutrients that help brain functioning, as well as lowering acidity levels in people who have routinely consumed a lot of alcohol or who have previously had a high sugar diet. This helps accelerate weight loss on the stomach and you can use this oil instead of butter by using it in your dishes and it can also be used in beverages and soups.

The Benefits of Fresh Pure Water

An important part of weight loss is choosing the right kind of drinks, as this is just as important as giving your body the right types of fats. Sports drinks, even low-calorie ones, can be tempting to consume as they boast to give you optimal hydration. However these actually do more harm than good when it comes to your efforts to drop pounds. This is because they are packed with a lot of sweeteners and sodium, so with a lot of food colouring and unhealthy sugars added they actually detrimental to what you're trying to achieve. Taking this into account, there is no better alternative than pure fresh water. And although some people like to say that water is too plain on the taste buds, you can easily add a slice of lemon or lime to dramatically change the flavour. Another way to increase your metabolism and regulate your blood pressure can be to add a few sprinkles of cayenne pepper to a tall grass and warm or cold water.

Amazingly, drinking green tea instead of coffee, as long as it is unsweetened, can actually give you as much as five pounds of weight loss in one week. So when you find it hard to shed those last few pounds take this into consideration for its possibly drastic positive

outcome. When it comes to caffeine in general, it is a good idea to heavily limit your intake. This includes all sodas, including diet soda as this has been proven to be just as bad for your body is the full sugar types, so to make the most of your workout and get the best results, go for pure fruit juice. Similarly to low-fat milk, you can consume several ounces of these per day and they will help add useful nutrients to your diet. It's fine to have one coffee in the morning - just go easy on the amount of sugar and cream that you have with it.

Why Snacking Can Help You In The Long-Run

It may be hard to believe, but dark chocolate is actually good for you. In fact, it is recommended as part of your regular walking for weight loss program as it can dramatically boost your serotonin levels. It's a guilt-free way to indulge in a tasty snack, whilst reducing your food cravings, therefore helping to diet in the long-run. So it's true that some of the most beneficial foods are some of the most tasty. So, denying your sweet tooth of chocolate entirely is actually worse for you overall as it has been proven that people who eat dark chocolate tend to eat a lot less than those that deny themselves of it entirely. It just goes to show that adding powerful nutrients can have its good moments. So when you feel lacking in motivation when it comes to your power walking for weight loss plan, an easy and quick way to get back your drive and lift your spirits is to indulge in a couple of rich squares of dark - keeping your hunger at bay in the process.

www.ingramcontent.com/pod-product-compliance
Lightning Source LLC
Chambersburg PA
CBHW061944280526
45787CB00004B/1724